How to Lose Weight Easily

and

Free Yourself From Diets Forever

Michael Hadfield

Michael Hadfield

Previously published in 2011 on Kindle

Contents

Introduction

Have you ever seen a fat lion? I haven't. I'm a keen watcher of wildlife programs and a frequent visitor to the local zoo and it seems to me that lions have it easy – in fact they appear to be in possession of the ultimate in weight control. They do an awful lot of lounging around in the sunshine. When they get hungry they go and kill something; eat it till they've had enough; and then go and lounge around some more. Every now and then they go for a wander down to the local waterhole for a drink, followed by a bit more lounging until next time they feel hungry.

So they eat as much as they want, don't seem to exercise that much, and maintain just the right weight. But then, when you think about it, a fat lion is going to have more than a bit of trouble jumping on the back of a wildebeest, or chasing after a zebra. Can you imagine it – a big, overweight, wobbly lion getting puffed after 30 yards of running after dinner, giving up, and just lying down for a rest? Wouldn't be fat for long would he?

So you see that there is a self-regulating mechanism occurring here. Not true of those slim lions in zoos though. They don't get to do much running or killing. Dinner is tossed over the fence every day – but they still stay slim. Then, I guess, someone is controlling how much they get, so maybe we should ignore caged animals while we look for an easy and comfortable way to lose weight.

So am I suggesting that in order to lose weight you should move to Africa and chase wildebeest for lunch?

Of course not. But what I am suggesting is that lions don't have to think about food in order to remain slim. All lions do is what comes naturally and then it happens anyway. So the first step is to consider that being slim is normal and natural, and so anything imposed upon you in the way of things like diets is most unlikely to provide you with a long-term solution to healthy weight loss.

On a more serious note - one of the big problems with rapid weight loss is the sudden release of toxins into the blood stream. Participants in a scientific research program who lost large amounts of weight over a short period of time had blood serum levels of 6 toxins 50% higher than those who had lost no weight. The solution offered in this book takes this into account.

You see, much of the food we eat, unless we are fortunate enough to enjoy a totally organic diet, is loaded with chemical pollutants. Some are sprayed on the food deliberately, or applied to the soil, or injected into the livestock, others just end up in our drinking water or sea food. In small quantities our bodies can just about handle these chemicals, but they are fat soluble, so if you are overeating and depositing fat the toxins get locked up in the fat cells – temporarily out of harm's way.

When you lose weight rapidly, these toxins are released in much higher quantities than normal into the blood stream – effectively poisoning you and putting a heavy load on organs, like the liver, to deal with the problem.

This book shows you how to make sure weight is lost at a healthy rate and doesn't involve you in any diets or restrictive eating practices. It is a much more natural system that allows you to lose weight easily and safely in a way that is not only sustainable, but leaves you feeling totally in control of your eating – rather than having your eating in control of you.

Michael Hadfield

1. The Wrong Trousers

In this book I hope to show you that losing weight does not need to be difficult. In fact, I intend to demonstrate that the reason you have found it so difficult to keep the weight off - even after you've successfully managed to lose it - is *The Diet* itself. This book isn't about rapid weight loss. Rapid weight loss is seriously damaging to your health and well-being. My intention is to show you that you can make small changes, changes that you can easily adapt to, that will make a big difference to your relationship with food. These easy changes will result in gentle, but permanent weight loss.

Diets actually make you fat and I've discovered that losing weight is a much more complicated issue than just watching how many calories you eat. In fact focusing on calories is just a distraction that prevents long-term success.

I will show you how you've been lied to and misled over the years and how what you've been taught is actually causing the difficulties you are experiencing in trying to lose weight.

Just so you know, I'm not someone who's been slim all his life trying to tell you how to lose excess weight. Way back around 1979 after having had a 34" waist since I reached adulthood, I suddenly found myself 3st (42lbs) overweight. Suddenly might seem an odd way to describe finding an extra 42lbs on a body, but because my weight was totally stable I rarely weighed myself and thought the increased waistline was not that significant, just a product of getting older. It was standing on the scales one day that made me realise just how much weight I'd added.

What happened was this. I couldn't drive back then so I went everywhere by bus and train - that meant walking to bus stops and train stations. I also cycled for pleasure. Then I got a job 32 miles away which entailed about three hours travelling each way by public transport (4 buses and a train). So I bought a motorcycle. I went from walking 5-6 miles a day to sitting on a motorcycle. That's where the weight came from. Nothing else had changed.

As soon as I realised what had happened I decided I needed to do something about it. Now this was in the days before the internet when information wasn't so readily available. I'd heard about diets and they didn't seem much fun so I made some decisions based around what I wanted, and what I intuitively knew to be right. Mostly I wanted to lose the weight. After that I mostly wanted not to be hungry (this seemed to be the major problem with diets and the reason I didn't want to do that). Then I wanted to eat what I wanted if I wanted to. That seemed pretty straightforward.

So here's what I did.

Breakfast remained the same, but I needed to get some exercise back into my day and the only time I really had available was a 30 minute lunch break, so I decided to use that. There was a park 5 minutes walk from the office so I did a fast walk around there every day. That was just about two miles. That left me a problem - lunch.

Where did I fit that in? This was the only major change I made. I stopped having sandwiches. I just took an apple and ate it while I was working. Surprisingly, I found that the apple satisfied me. I soon got used to just having that and it left me with a really nice appetite by the time I got home for dinner. Dinner was just the same as it always was. Then I cut out supper, which was usually a couple of slices of toast and jam. This was a habit from childhood. And although I missed it for a few days, what I found was that I felt really pleased with myself the next morning for not having given in to temptation. The only other real changes I made were that I decided that if I need to fill up I'd fill up on potatoes and wholemeal bread (I used to eat white bread). The reasoning being that the fibre in the wholemeal bread would swell up in my stomach and cause a fuller feeling than an equivalent amount of white bread. Potatoes were just a cheap, bulky, healthy vegetable full of vitamins and minerals.

That's pretty much it. I never went hungry. If any of the changes I made left me feeling hungry any time, I ate. It was no big deal. If I went out I'd have coffee and cake. If someone offered me stuff I'd enjoy it and not feel even slightly guilty. I suppose mostly I didn't make an issue of it. I just decided what I was going to do and did it. It wasn't anything to do with anyone else, and anytime I didn't want to do it I didn't. But there was never any beating up or feeling guilty. I recognised the pointlessness of all of that.

Now just in case you are wondering, this book is not 'The Apple for Lunch and a Walk Round the Park' diet, though, now I think about it, that might be a good book title and a wonderful new fad diet. If only I was a celebrity, I could probably make a fortune out of that. Anyway I lost the 40 odd pounds in whatever time it took and it was no big deal. I never returned to a 34" waist but I was quite happy with 36" where it stayed until very recently.

I bought some new trousers without realising they had a well-hidden expanding waist, so my weight snuck up without me realising it. A tightening waistline is what I use nowadays to tell me to make some changes. It was only when these expanding trousers wore out and I bought a replacement pair (without an expanding waist) that I found I couldn't fasten them because I'd grown too fat. That's when I realised what had happened.

Since I've been working with weight loss for quite a while, I figured out that it can be even easier now than it was for me way back in '79. So I used this as an opportunity to test my stuff out on me. I like to use me as a guinea pig for what I teach, just to make sure it works. I'm pretty set in my ways so if something works for me it'll probably work for you. Although I've been working with weight loss for 14 years I only know that what I do works because my clients tell me that. Up until now I've had no personal experience of it.

At the time of writing, I've lost 12lbs, so far. Not quite sure when I started because I had a target weight in mind, knew I would reach it, and wasn't too bothered how long it took. I've lost this weight just using what I teach here. But it doesn't just work for me; it also works extremely well for others too.

This is what my latest client said to me, as she was leaving, after her final treatment visit a couple of days ago...

"I feel like my eating is under control, now."

Michael Hadfield

2. What You Really, Really, Want!

Of course, what you really want is to lose all of your excess weight right now - isn't it? And you'd like me to tell you how to work that trick, even though you know that it's impossible. But that doesn't stop you wanting and wishing for that miracle. And if I could get rid of all 40lbs of it by the time you set off on holiday in 4 weeks time, you'd want to get started straight away. Unfortunately I can't do any of *that* for you. I can't even help you to get rid of all your excess weight in the next 6 weeks using some mystical, magical crash diet eating some amazing sludge that not only fills you up but also meets every single one of your body's vitamin, mineral and calorie requirements and makes you feel so bloated that you'll never want to eat again.

We've all been taken in by that sort of nonsense. We're taken in because it promises what we most want in the world - to be attractive, and confident, and loved, and it promises to hand it over to us almost as fast as we hand over our money to its purveyors. But the main attraction of that sort of gunk is that in two or three or four or six weeks, the problem is solved. Six weeks of hell, go on holiday looking slim and gorgeous, come home, and get straight back to eating all the stuff that piles the weight back on, until you repeat the same thing with a different Gunk next year. Aren't you tired of all of that? Wouldn't you like to lose weight just one more time, do it properly and discover that you can keep it off and still eat what you want?

If you really are serious about losing weight then read on and find out what works and what doesn't and the reasons why. But before we get on to that let's have a look at what you really, really want. I've created a list of popular reasons for wanting to be slimmer. See how many of them apply to you.

- Do you want to be your ideal size and shape?

- Do you want to be gorgeous?

- Do you want to be able to move around easily and bend freely?

- Do you want to walk and climb stairs without effort?

- Do you want to run around and play with your children or grandchildren?

- Do you want to buy the clothes you love instead of the ones they have in your size?

- Do you want to feel attractive again?

- Do you want members of the opposite sex to look at you – in a good way?

- Do you also want all of that without having to make any changes to your eating habits?

- Do you want to eat *what* you want?

- Do you want to eat *when* you want?

If you go out for a meal with friends do you want to select whatever you fancy and enjoy every last mouthful – regardless of calories, or carbs, or fat? And when it's time for dessert do you want to be able to choose the gooiest, creamiest, sweetest, most delicious looking offering on the menu totally regardless of how full you already feel?

You want all this, yet you believe it to be unattainable and so you just give up - if not today, then tomorrow, if not tomorrow then next week. Sooner or later you just give up and the pounds keep piling on until you need to shift up another dress size or trouser size and then you start up the treadmill all over again.

Sound familiar?

What diets do is create a battleground within your mind where you have a set of rules to apply (carbs, Calories, syns, points, grams of fat…) and that set of rules sets up a psychological resistance (no one likes being told what to do) that causes you to want to defy the rules while at the same time understanding that it is counter-productive. It's a no-win situation where food becomes the Enemy, eating is always a battle and hunger is frequently around. But more on that later, because first, I need to tell you a little bit more about me and how I can help you.

Michael Hadfield

3. Who Am I?

Since you've probably never heard of me I should really explain why I'm qualified to help you lose all of that excess weight. I told you earlier about my own personal experiences with being overweight. I explained how I solved my weight problem in ways that were acceptable to me, rather than following a set of rules that someone else had created and that probably wouldn't work. With my first attempt at weight loss, I lost 42lbs based on a system of my own devising, and kept it off for over 25 years. Since then I became a therapist and found myself specialising in weight loss and the frequently connected areas of confidence, self-esteem, stress and anxiety. I like to help people discover they can be successful despite what they believe about themselves and regardless of how many times they might have tried and failed. I change lives. I give people their freedom to be who they want to be. I teach people how to think differently about their problems, how to change their worldview, and how to get what they want, and then I usually use hypnosis to reinforce the message and make it much, much easier to make the necessary changes...

"When I came to see you I was around 16 stone 10lbs (234 lbs). I am pleased to tell you that I have lost weight and am currently 13 stone (182lbs), so I have gone below my target weight. I feel that I have done myself proud, and I doubt I would have been able to do this without your help"

JD

…and when people who are serious about losing weight come to me for help, when they follow my guidance – they usually lose weight, easily and effortlessly…

"I lost 28lbs and easily kept it off. I feel good and am enjoying life much more"

AS

…and it stays off.

So if you are finding that Life is just a battle with food & weight and all that happens when you diet is that you end up thinking all the time about food. Then you need to be careful. Continuing to read this may just end all of that for you - forever.

4. Here's What I Can Do For You.

I've written this book to help you lose weight. So if you are serious about losing weight and prepared to make some small, easy changes, then I am certain that this book will help you to get what you want. But you need to want it enough, and you need to believe that it is possible for you to lose the weight you want to lose.

I had a call the other evening from a potential client wanting some information about the weight loss program I offer. As I was talking to her and mentioning some of the things I touched on above, I could hear her enthusiasm growing as I spoke to her. She recognised that she was finally talking to someone who truly understood the problems she had encountered in the past when trying to lose weight.

I explained to her that the key to success is determination.

That caused a little reticence, and I could *feel* her withdrawing from the conversation, so I explained what I meant by determination. Determination isn't the same as failing and then trying again; then failing again and trying again, and still failing. Determination is knowing that success is inevitable because you are going to keep going until you arrive. It's just making a decision that you know you are going to stick to. In the story about my current episode of weight loss I said I wasn't sure how long I'd been doing this for. The duration wasn't important because I was determined to lose the excess.

For me determination is just an inner knowing that I will reach the target. With that, I don't need a timescale. In fact I believe a timescale is counter-productive. Once you accept that success is inevitable, you cannot fail. Once you keep a goal permanently in mind, the past is irrelevant. All that matters is whether or not what you are doing right now is consistent with your goal. If it isn't you have the choice to change it. And, in a nutshell, that's exactly what I'm going to teach you how to do.

If losing weight the old way was easy you'd surely have done it already. But you keep on doing it and failing. You might lose weight and keep it off for a while, but sooner or later it returns and you find yourself back on the hamster wheel. And of course there's all that food you really, really enjoy but is so fattening and so delicious and it would be just a horrible life sentence never to be able to eat that stuff again.

And you always want to eat. And you've failed so many times you have almost no expectation of success. You want someone to wave a magic wand and make it all go away. I know it's easier to believe in magic than to believe in yourself, and a lot of people who come to me for help really want magic. Sometimes the results are *like* magic, but most of the time it's the two of us working together to achieve the desired results.

So, knowing that I usually achieve the desired result, what if I told you that you *can* lose weight? What if I told you that you *can* keep it off? What if I told you that you can not only do this, but also eat what you want when you want?

If you are as sceptical as I am then you probably think that's too good to be true and would be very wary. I don't blame you - it certainly sounds like some sort of scam.

You know what they say... if it's too good to be true - it probably isn't.

It only sounds too good to be true because the difficulty is not where you think it is. What would be too good to be true would be if I were telling you that you can carry on exactly as you always have done and I will still help you to lose weight. But that isn't what I'm saying. I'm saying I know how to make the necessary changes you need to make in order to lose weight and those changes will not only be changes in your eating patterns, but also changes in your thought patterns about food.

But, and this is most important, those changes do not need you to ban any particular foods. And because there is no ban on any particular foods we banish cravings completely. We completely eliminate the battleground, so there is no battle. You will not suffer. You can eat what you want, but you will eat less of it and still feel satisfied if you follow my guidance. I need to stress that the 'eating less' isn't any kind of a trick, or a way to turn this into a calorie-reduced diet. The eating less is discovering that most of the food you eat is eaten unconsciously and not enjoyed - or even noticed most of the time. I encourage you to eat consciously, enjoying and savouring every mouthful until your body tells you that it has eaten sufficiently - for now. I encourage you to eat when you are hungry. I certainly do. While I was losing those 12lbs I mentioned earlier, I enjoyed cake, chocolate biscuits, chips, apple pie, crisps and other forbidden foods. There was no deprivation and so no craving. In fact I'm finding, as I continue with this process, that I'm experiencing a loss of interest in food. Life isn't about food. Life isn't about all the food you will miss if you attain and sustain a healthy weight. If food is your only pleasure, then you really need to start exploring other sources of creative stimulation and entertainment, because if that really is what your life revolves around then you may find it difficult (not impossible though) to release your attachment to it. If you've dragged a ball and chain around all your life, then freedom may make you feel uncomfortable and strangely light for a while.

That reminds me of a story I read about how they train elephants in India. If you want to picture in your mind something big and heavy, an elephant is a pretty good candidate. A full grown elephant, as I'm sure you realise, is a beast to be reckoned with and not an animal that a puny human could tell what to do. After all, when elephants get mad, they can pick up a person and dash them to the ground as though they were a rag doll. But elephants are animals that are trained for forestry work and their mahouts have little difficulty getting them to haul heavy logs, or anything else they want them to do. And do you know how they stop them from wandering off at night? They fasten a stake to the ground and tie the elephant's leg to it with a bit of rope. The interesting thing is that if the elephant just walked away, the rope would snap, or the stake would pull out of the ground. The stake and rope do not actually secure the elephant, because they are nowhere near strong enough. What makes the rope and stake work is an idea in the elephant's mind.

The mahout starts with the elephant when it is very young, and ties it to a stake. The stake and rope are sufficiently strong to prevent a baby elephant from getting away. But the baby elephant pulls and struggles against the restraint until it eventually learns that it is a waste of time. Then the elephant gives up. It knows that it is pointless pulling against the rope - so it stops. And it *never* pulls against the rope again. The elephant grows up, but doesn't realise that rope and stake don't. It doesn't continue to test them as it gets bigger. It believes it is not free and behaves accordingly. As soon as the rope is placed around its leg when work is finished for the day, the elephant just stays put.

This is a demonstration of the power of conditioning. You can experience something in childhood and believe it to be true for the rest of your life. You can feel overwhelmed, or believe that something is impossible, and that belief can be so powerful that you never bother to test it out and see if it is still true for you. How much of your inability to control your eating is down to you constantly telling yourself that you can't? If this is true for you, you might consider changing that message slightly and just start telling yourself 'I don't know how to control my eating yet?'

When you approach losing weight the right way – the way I'm teaching you – you may discover that it can be even easier than you thought. I believe it is possible for you to have what you want. I say this because, over the years, I have helped many people to have what they wanted. There is one thing I need to stress though. If you are in your 30's or 40's or 50's and very overweight it is unlikely that you will return to being the sylph-like 16 year old you once were. So be realistic in your aims. If you are realistic you can do it and you can succeed. If you are unrealistic with your target weight then all you do is set yourself up for failure and disappointment. So, aim initially to lose 10lbs or 20lbs (or to drop one clothes size) - even if you want to eventually lose much more than that. That way you can enjoy success when you hit your target and you can enjoy *that* success and all it brings with it. Then, knowing that you now know how to achieve a target weight, or clothes size, you can set another target of 5lbs or 10lbs and succeed at that. When you break this process into manageable chunks you enjoy success after success after success and the whole weight loss process just becomes an enjoyable game. A game where you win every single time you play.

Sound good?

Are you ready to succeed?

Okay, so now we get down to the nitty gritty - what exactly do you have to do that's different from everything you've tried in the past and how will it help you to lose those excess pounds?

5. Why Diets Don't Work

...and you keep hoping they will.

I'm going to tell you about the problems with diets, why they don't work, why they actually make you fat, and how I can help you to lose weight without dieting.

But first let's have a little look at insanity.

Insanity

"Doing the same thing over and over again but expecting different results."

Rita Mae Brown (Sudden Death 1983)

'Try harder' - have you ever heard that one. It's a powerful subliminal message programmed into most of us. If your test score isn't high enough then you must *try harder*. If you fail at anything then clearly you didn't *try hard enough*.

No matter how hard I tried I couldn't win races at school because everyone else was faster than I was and I got asthma when I exercised. Trying harder didn't make any difference. A pair of rocket-propelled shoes might. If the phone is broken, pressing the buttons harder won't make it work. If you have difficulty retaining information then stuffing more in isn't going to fix your memory. Trying harder is just doing the same thing over and over again.

What works is a totally different approach to the problem.

Rocket-propelled shoes, repairing the phone, learning Tony Buzan's excellent techniques on how to improve your memory will all create the desired results (well, possibly not the rocket-propelled shoes, but I don't want to be too serious here).

Although diet-free weight loss works without diets (and by diets I mean some mechanism for restricting food intake based around calories or food-types) you are still required to make changes. So you have to be prepared for some change. The changes I ask you to make are easy, and most importantly – sustainable. The reason they are sustainable is because diet-free weight loss helps you to change your mind so that you find it easier to make choices that are consistent with your long-term goal of reducing your weight and changing your body-shape and size.

First recognise and acknowledge that you have a problem. And if this sounds like AA it's not deliberate. Acknowledging that you have a problem is the first step towards freedom. It is the taking of responsibility. Responsibility is not blame because you are not the cause. But you are the cure. You are the cure because you are the only one who can fix this. You don't have to fix it on your own. I'll help you and guide you through that process. But you do have to recognise that whatever its cause, you have a problem NOW that you want to fix.

Before I show you how to fix it I'd like to give you a feel for the scale of this problem that you are a part of. The problem is a social one much more than it is a personal one. But society isn't going to fix it either. There's only one person who can fix it – and that's you. But because it is a huge problem within the society that you are a part of, there is a lot of pressure from outside of you to conform to what everyone else is doing. This makes learning techniques of weight control a lonely journey most of the time. But rest assured – you are not alone.

Most of the dieters I talk to see themselves as to blame for their own failure. It's really important to know that you were programmed to fail. The diet industry's survival depends upon your failure. If diets worked, you would only have to diet once.

Consider this…

When something works, you do it and enjoy success.

When something doesn't work you do it…

…and do it…

…and do it…

…and do it…

Remember the quote about the definition of insanity? Doing the same thing over and over yet expecting different results.

What the Diet Industry does is to convince you that you are the one who isn't doing it right, and then they get you to do it again, and again, and again. Every year at Resolution Time just after the Christmas Holiday, and again in the spring, the serial dieters return to the fat-clubs like Weight-Watchers and Slimming World and greet each other like the old friends they are. It's a great social outing and nice to be with people who have the same problem as you. Even nicer to see the few who have a serious obesity problem because it makes our 30 lbs of excess weight seem almost slim.

I'm not knocking these organisations (well maybe a little bit - but good-naturedly). They perform a service and if what they sell is what you want, then have lots of it. It's just not what I do, and from what I can see, it doesn't create lasting change. I know that because a lot of the people who end up in my consulting room, desperately wanting to find some way of losing weight that works, have already tried those places. It also seems appropriate to understand that what you are dealing with is not a small local group but a massive business. Weight Watchers 2010 revenue was $1,452,000,000. Their assets are valued at just over $1 billion. Nothing wrong with being a successful company, but successful companies, in my experience, seem to be more about making money than making a difference. If you were in charge of a company making $1.5 billion a year out of people wanting to lose weight, would you want to cure all the fat people or would you find some way to keep them coming back for more. From a business point of view it's very much cheaper to keep a customer than to attract a new one. The only way you can keep an overweight customer is to keep your customer overweight. After all, a big business answers first of all to its shareholders. Shareholders need nice dividends and an increasing share price to provide a worthwhile return on their investment. I'm just me, I don't have any shareholders, and, unfortunately, I always have to attract new customers because I keep 'fixing' them.

If diets worked, you would diet once and no one could make that much money out of you. In order to maintain the massive revenue and lifestyles of those in the weight loss industry, diets have to be designed to fail to keep weight off while giving you short-term success so you keep coming back believing that you just need to try harder (remember insanity) and that it's really your fault because you didn't do it well enough.

You only failed because the system is designed to fail. It's just more psychological conditioning where the use of a reward (the weight loss) is connected with attendance at these 'classes'. What this does is program you to engage in the *attend a weight club* behaviour whenever you want to lose weight - without ever questioning the fact that the weight has returned and the weight club only created short-term results.

"I estimate I spent, you know, tens of thousands - maybe $100,000 - on different kinds of diet products, diet services, and I was still fat."

Wendy Shanker

Diets make you... think about food... feel deprived... and crave what you can't have.

"One failure of most diet plans is that people get hungry and quit."

Frank M. Sacks M.D. (dietary expert)

21% of dieters give up in less than 2 months. 45% of dieters give up in less than 12 months. So you can see that about 1 in 5 dieters only stick to the diet for two months ...and almost half give up in less than a year.

What I'd like you to consider is that this is a game - a game where you have been manipulated and lied to for the benefit of others.

A game you can't win.

The revenue of the US weight loss industry in 2010 was

$60,000,000,000

Forecasts for the Global weight loss industry for 2014 suggest that its revenue will exceed

$586,300,000,000

That's half a trillion dollars!

6. It Says so on the Telly so it Must be Good...

With half a trillion dollars at stake do you think they really care as long as they can continue to sell you small meals in fancy packets for three times the price of twice as much? I remember, from the 60's, a product called Nimble. I don't think it's made any more. It was dieters' bread. I think the advert claimed it was half the calories per slice. The loaf itself was half the size of a standard loaf, and as you would expect, more expensive. The slices were also about half the size of a standard loaf. It seemed to me it had half the calories per slice because the slice was half the size - in other words, it was just bread. But it was bread in a fancy packet with a big advertising budget (involving hot air balloon TV ads to emphasise its lightness, with a nimble and attractive young actress riding in the balloon) - a total rip-off, in my humble opinion.

Now look at what happens when you try to lose weight using those traditional methods that weight loss product promoters, and TV ads, encourage you to use.

Food is restricted.

Food supply is limited.

The most desirable foods are banned.

This causes CRAVING.

This causes Food Obsession.

Food effectively becomes something with a limited and controlled supply because that's what you tell yourself when you limit calorie intake and put certain foods off limits or allow yourself only small quantities. The BIG mistake is to think that just eating less is the solution. It Isn't! That's the reason you end up craving. Not because you are hungry. Not because there's anything wrong with you. Just because you are pretending that food is in short supply. ... and the food in the shortest supply is the food you most enjoy.

Research shows that diets make you hungry and create powerful cravings for things like sugars and fats.

There is also that deprived feeling of everyone else can have it so why can't I? This is especially true when you are eating out with friends and see them enjoying luscious, creamy, chocolate-covered goop.

"The more we endure cycles of dieting, the more our bodies become trained to seek out food, slow down vital functions and conserve body fat. In the forest, sweetness was nature's way of telling early humans that fruit was safe to eat."

"In evolutionary terms, the human body cannot distinguish between dieting and famine. We are hard-wired to respond to the threat of an insecure food supply by retaining body fat rather than burning it off, just as camels are biologically designed to store fat in humps to survive forays in the desert."

Geoffrey Cannon author of Dieting Makes You Fat.

Now it's time for a slight change of direction.

7. Diets Focus on Food.

Let's imagine for a minute that you are a chocolate lover and I tell you NOT to think about chocolate. Take a few moments to not think about chocolate and then when you haven't thought about chocolate for a minute or so, come back.

What were you thinking about – chocolate?

And if you think I am somehow playing mind games with you rather than trying to help you to understand how your mind works, then you might be deliberately not-thinking about chocolate. But, realise this, in order to not think about something you still have to hold the idea of it in your mind in order to know what it is you are not thinking about. And even if you have convinced yourself you aren't thinking about chocolate – you will.

Because diets are about *not* doing this, and *not* doing that, you end up thinking about the thing you are not supposed to do. You have to; otherwise habit would just have you doing it.

But what's the last thing you want to think about when you are dieting?

That's right, all of those foods you aren't allowed to eat any more.

Diets also focus on weight loss. What I'll show you later is that weight loss is not fat loss and weight loss is not changing your body shape the way you want.

Michael Hadfield

8. State of Mind.

Being slimmer is not just about calories. Being slim is a state of mind. If there is no change in attitudes to food, eating, and self, then a diet will not succeed in bringing about permanent weight change.

Let me give you an example, simply from observing other people eating.

I was in Asda (the local Wal-mart owned supermarket) sitting in the sunshine and warmth of the conservatory café enjoying a cup of their excellent coffee, along with a good book, when I realised that most of the customers in the café were more than a little overweight.

Interesting, I thought, and did a quick count. 8 overweight, 3 about average, and two slim. Then I noticed what they were eating. Now, I have to say that Asda is typical cafeteria food – chips, sausage, fried eggs, greasy looking lasagne (that's just the liquefying cheese though), meat pie… Good variety, but I don't remember seeing any salad. I had some kind of cake there once and it wasn't good cake.

So you can see that if you wanted to eat healthily you'd simply go somewhere else. I noticed plates piled high, and then cleaned – with one exception. The slim people were a couple with a baby. The young lady had had a plate of chips and other stuff and she had finished her meal. She was enjoying her conversation with her partner and keeping an eye on baby, but about three quarters of the meal was still on the plate (clearly finished and pushed to one side) and no attention was being paid to all that 'wasted' food.

This reminded me of something I'd read, it said slim people think about food in a way that's quite different from the way overweight people think about food. Slim people don't have better metabolisms or anything genetic to keep them that way. They simply see food as fuel and when they've had sufficient they've had sufficient and nothing would cause them to eat any more – no matter how much is left on the plate, or how attractive the gateaux or cheesecake appear.

For a slim person food has no personality; it has no power; it has no way to affect how they feel. If they feel good they feel good. If they feel low they feel low. Food just doesn't enter into it. Does that mean they don't enjoy what they eat – no! It means they enjoy it fully while they are eating it, but when they are full they stop. They don't then mourn the loss of the pleasure left on the plate. They see it for what it is – a congealing mess that if anyone was presented with as it is, would go straight in the bin.

Think about that. The difference between overweight and slim could be nothing more than the way you think about food.

Diet-free weight loss works on changing the attitudes, beliefs, eating patterns, and behaviours that keep you overweight. It allows you to change gently, and therefore, permanently - if that is what you want?

Diet-Free Weight Loss focuses on you feeling good. Because there are no restrictions you will almost certainly find that any obsessive thoughts about food, which you may have experienced in the past, will gradually dissipate. They dissipate as your body/mind adapts to the changes. As your eating patterns become normal, your weight reduces gradually and naturally.

One of the biggest problems with diet and weight loss organisations is that they lie to you. They con you into believing that you are losing fat. Weight-loss is not fat loss.

Muscle tissue burns more Calories (an incredible 30 times more) than fat tissue. So in times of food shortage, muscle tissue is the first to go because it is the biggest threat to survival. Reduced muscle mass means lower Calorie requirements therefore greater chance of survival.

"Diets do not lead to sustained weight loss or health benefits for the majority of people. You can initially lose 5 to 10% of your weight on any number of diets, but then the weight comes back."

Traci Mann, Psychologist
University of California, Los Angeles

When normal eating is eventually restored, you have altered the ratio of fat/muscle so metabolic rate is lower. All that repeated dieting does is lower metabolism and increase the ratio of fat to muscle. Because metabolism is lowered, it's harder to burn off what you eat and so fat deposition increases. Weight loss is almost entirely down to muscle loss. Muscle is denser than body fat so body shape does not change much, even though pounds are being lost. You can end up at a 'normal' weight but with a very high percentage of body fat. When normal eating is restored, fat deposition is also restored and the situation worsens. This is why yo-yo dieting is a major health risk.

Dieting turns muscle to fat.

"We found that the majority of people regained all the weight, plus more. Sustained weight loss was found only in a small minority of participants, while complete weight regain was found in the majority."

Traci Mann, Psychologist
University of California, Los Angeles

... and to prove it you'll find that the vast majority of people who diet are fatter two years later than if they had never bothered trying to lose weight.

9. Diets Screw You Up

A diet causes long-term weight gain.

Every time you diet it gets harder to achieve the same results.

Every time you diet you lose a little more faith in yourself and your ability to succeed in life.

Diets are seriously unhealthy things to do to your body. You *can* lose weight if you make small changes that become a normal natural part of your life. Diet-Free Weight Loss is not a quick fix, it's a permanent change. And because it's a permanent change it has to be comfortable – otherwise it would be unsustainable. Consequently, weight loss is slow.

Would you be happy to lose 50lbs?

If you lost as little as a pound a week (this would not be entertained by most serial dieters) that's 50lbs in a year. That's as much weight as most people want to lose.

...or 100lbs?

If you lost that tiny amount for two years that's 100lbs (I'm giving you a couple of weeks off for Christmas and holidays). If you could do that for 4 years there probably wouldn't be anything left of you. So you see it's not the amount that's important, or the speed with which you lose weight. When you make the choice to get off the diet treadmill and make small sustainable changes to your eating habits and your relationship with food, you make the choice to allow your body, naturally, to slim down. You don't need to make a big deal out of it.

Another benefit is that if you lose just a pound a week then by the time you reach your target weight, and body shape, you will be in total control of your eating, and eating will be a pleasure for you.

10. Change

"If you do what you've always done, you'll get what you've always gotten."

"The past doesn't equal the future."

Anthony Robbins author of Unlimited Power

One thing I must tell you though, is that in order for you to have what you want – something must change.

Obviously if nothing changes there can be no different outcomes.

Think about that for a moment

If nothing changes, how can you expect different results?

In order to achieve consistent results I focus on small changes, because small changes are easy. It is a diet-free system. There are absolutely no food restrictions. However, I encourage you to make healthy choices - but that's just because healthy choices make it much easier to: lose weight; stay fit & healthy; feel satisfied after a meal; and maintain a positive mood state.

If you follow my guidance I can help you to not only make those changes, but also to enjoy well-deserved success.

So how do you get this?

It is very, very simple.

All you need to do is to *realistically* decide on either your target weight or a target clothes size. Personally I feel that aiming for a clothes size makes the process easier, but that has to be your choice depending on whether or not weekly weighing motivates or distresses you when change isn't happening in the direction you want or as fast as you want. This is a really important decision for you to make, because this process is a slow and gentle re-education of your attitudes and relationship with food you may well find that some weeks you put on a pound or two and others you lose them. If you understand that this is natural and normal that's okay - go for weekly weighing just so you stay motivated. If the slightest weight increase makes you want to give up and think this isn't working then aim for a clothes size reduction and steer clear of the scales. But whatever you choose make a genuine commitment to yourself to stay with the process until you achieve and maintain either your weight or size. By that time the changes you have made and sustained will be second nature to you, so maintaining your weight will become quite natural and you probably won't even think about it.

I remember, quite a few years ago, a client came to me for some help with weight loss. When she came back a week later for the second session, she'd gained two pounds in weight. A lot of people probably wouldn't have come back for the second session after a result like that. But when she returned for the third session, after a another week of progress, she reported a weight loss of 6lbs.

In order to succeed all you need is to be serious about losing weight. You need to understand that as long as the trend is downwards, you can enjoy short-term increases without worrying. You need to have stopped playing the dieting game. And you need to have a goal weight or size that you know is achievable for you.

This is a change that takes just a few weeks to master, but is easily sustainable, it is a change of your whole relationship with food, a change that will allow you to get more pleasure from what you eat while steadily dropping those pounds.

I believe that I can help you to lose weight and that I can do it more easily than you thought possible.

The Diet-Free Weight Loss System works because it solves all the problems that diets don't, it is long-term sustainable without any discomfort, and you don't have to spend the rest of your life fighting with food. Diet-Free Weight Loss focuses on: small, sustainable changes; no food restrictions; no more diets; no public humiliation at weigh-ins, no Guilt.

That last point is a biggy. Guilt probably puts on more pounds of fat than anything else. Slimming World even have a book out called 'Slimming World Free Foods: Guilt-free food whenever you're hungry' - the very strong implication being that there *are* foods you *should* feel guilty about when you eat. This, in my opinion, is absolute tosh. Eat what you want. Just learn how to stop when you are satisfied, rather than when you are finished.

While on a diet have you ever experienced feeling a bit low? Maybe it's just that the weight isn't shifting fast enough? Maybe you are fed-up eating lettuce or feeling hungry? Or maybe you've just had a bad day at work, or a disagreement with your partner who is now enjoying himself in the pub? Then, bored, upset, or just fed-up, you find yourself fighting the urge to eat and then finally giving in. After you've eaten you realise the food has done nothing to change your mood state. Then you feel guilty because you failed with your diet or guilty because you couldn't say no and you feel utterly powerless so your mood drops even lower and before you know it you're back in the kitchen finding another snack...

That's guilt.

You can safely ignore it. Guilt is always about the past not about the present. You cannot change the past. Even if you're sitting down for your fourth snack as your mood sinks lower and lower, recognise the only point of action you have is the present. You can only stop eating what you are eating. You cannot stop eating what you've already eaten. You cannot stop eating what you are planning on not eating tomorrow. So forget about it, it doesn't help, and as we've seen, worrying about it only makes the situation worse. Eat what you eat. Don't eat what you don't eat. And, whichever it is, be ok with it. If you don't like the choices you've made, then make a different choice right now *in this moment*. It's no good making a choice now for tomorrow evening when you are bored or sad or fed-up and watching some mindless nonsense on TV. Make that choice tomorrow. Do it NOW, or don't do it. Saying you'll do it tomorrow is just an excuse to prevent feeling guilty now. The only choice you can ever impact is the one you are in the process of making. Recognise this and refer all choices to your Master Intention (I want to be xxx lbs, or size xx) and decide which is going to make you happier, being slim, or eating now. I can guarantee that the only answer to this question is the achievement of your Master Intention.

Remember Kate Moss' words "Nothing tastes as good as skinny feels"

Now we both know we're not aiming for skinny, we are aiming for slimmer, but we understand the intent of that phrase and I strongly suggest you remember it and repeat it to yourself as often as temptation rears its head. No food eaten in a state of low mood will make you feel as good as achieving your target weight or size. It's always a simple choice and a simple question. What do I most want? If you are not actually hungry, then 'to eat' can never be the answer. What you almost certainly want is to feel good. If you feel bad and that's what is driving your thoughts towards food - recognise also that this is simply an evasion so you don't have to deal with looking at your life situation right now. I know many ways of improving mood states and not one of them requires putting anything in your mouth.

If you're still with me, and I hope you are because the solution isn't actually that difficult, here's what you have to do: accept that in order to lose weight something has to change; accept that nothing you have tried has worked long-term; recognise that past failure has no bearing on the present; and choose a target that is achievable.

Consider which is best... 30lbs lost forever, or 60lbs lost for 6 months and 80lbs put back on in the next 12.

11. Resistance is Futile

Let me tell you a story.

From the age of 9 until I was 20 my Dad worked for the biscuit company, Jacob's, based in Liverpool. One of the perks was access to the company shop and an unlimited supply of low-price biscuits. I did a summer job there once, loading biscuit lorries. That was after I'd finished sixth-form college and was waiting to start a degree course. I really liked that company shop.

But going back to when I was 9, I remember that in the bottom of our kitchen cupboard was a big silver metal tin full of unwrapped Jacobs Club chocolate biscuits - milk chocolate finger biscuits, dark chocolate finger biscuits, milk chocolate fruit biscuits, and that occasional joy when I bit into it and discovered there was no biscuit at all and it was just a biscuit-shaped solid bar of chocolate, mmm.... When it was finished another tin replaced it. Sometimes there were two of these tins. Quite often there were other biscuits in the cupboard as well and since Tobler were part of the same group there was frequently exotic Swiss chocolate there too.

There were no restrictions placed on eating the biscuits. My sister and I could just help ourselves whenever we wanted and have as many as we wanted. We both grew up slim and healthy. I was just about 6ft and 147lbs when I was 21 and I was still the same weight 5 years later. My excess weight didn't arrive until my late 20's but I've already told you about that and how I dealt with it. What I'd like you to do is to remember this story because I'm going to come back to it later. It is highly relevant to losing weight without dieting.

But before I do that I want to look at how our relationship with food gets screwed up in the first place.

12. The Training

As a society we have a slightly skewed relationship with food. Consider a typical young child's birthday party. Jelly, cake, ice cream – lots of gooey things. Lots of things full of sugar. Lots of those bright unnatural colours. And what do we give them to take away after they have already over-filled themselves? We give them a goody bag filled with chocolate and even more brightly coloured sugars and probably even a few leftovers from the party.

Don't we just *hate* to see good food go to waste?

When children are upset what happens. They are given chocolate, ice cream, or some brightly coloured sugars in an attempt to change their mood state. And it works – but not for the reason we think it does. I'll tell you that reason after I mention one or two other key pieces of information.

When we were good, or mastered some aspect of life that pleased our parents, we received a treat - that treat was frequently in the form of fat and sugar. If you are a parent you will be doing exactly the same with your children. I know I did with mine.

As an adult, celebrations are usually accompanied by lots of food and although, as adults, we tend not to tolerate quite such a high naked sugar content, and are not so attracted by bright colours, we still lap the sugar up when it's mixed with wheat, chocolate, and cream or some other fat.

So we grow up associating the very worst aspects of our diet with the very best things that happen to us in life – reaching goals, being loved, being cared for, and pleasing others.

So how can you possibly win at this weight loss game when life has distorted your view of food to such an extent that not having those kinds of food in your life makes it seem almost as if life is not worth living without them? The sense of deprivation is just so strong that it seems more powerful than we are.

13. The Lost Art of Letting Go.

I hope that you are now a lot clearer about how you managed to arrive at such a distorted and unhealthy relationship with food. Most people, if they find themselves in an unhealthy relationship, simply end it. It might not be easy. It might be heartbreaking, but they do it, and once it's done, after a few weeks they invariably feel better, lighter, and much more in control of their lives.

Now go back to thinking about those treats when you were upset. Those things our parents lovingly gave us in the hope that they would help us to feel better. It wasn't the thing that we got that made us feel better. It was the love for us that was being expressed with that gift. It was the attention. They made us feel better. And the other thing that I mentioned earlier... the treat was also a distraction, it made us think about the treat and not whatever it was that was causing the upset – and chances are, by the time we'd finished the treat, we'd forgotten about whatever it was that was upsetting us.

You see, that's one thing that young children are very good at – forgetting about upsets. Best friends can become worst enemies and best friends again all in the space of a few minutes. If you have young children, you'll know how unconcerned they are about bearing grudges or hanging on to their unhappy feelings. They recognise that they are just feelings and don't need to be hung on to - because they don't really mean anything. And they are much happier than the adults surrounding them who like to hang on to hurts, and slights, and grudges, and a whole stack of negative emotions. We adults like to nurture our negative emotions and make them last as long as we possibly can. We cultivate them and fertilise them and make sure they bear tons of fruit. Just to make ourselves miserable.

And what did our parents do when we felt miserable – they gave us fats and sugars and bright colours. And we felt better.

14. Food = Happiness

Ivan Pavlov was a Professor of Pharmacology (later Professor of Physiology) at the Military Medical Academy in St Petersburg, who in 1905 was studying reflex physiology. He trained dogs to salivate at things they associated with food, like the sound of a bell, or a white coat - rather than at the presence of food itself. It's called Classical Conditioning, and I've given you some examples of this already - remember the elephant. Think of this in terms of commercial breaks during TV programmes, or coffee breaks at work.

Another word for this is habit. But Pavlov also discovered that he could untrain his dogs just as easily as long as he did it deliberately and methodically. Habits can be broken.

But going back to our childhood training and how it affects us as adults - what do we do when we feel miserable? We go seeking those fats and sugars because we have this crazy idea that they will make us feel better because that's what happened when Mum or Dad or Auntie or Nan, gave us fats and sugars when we were little. We fail to make the connection that it was attention and love and distraction that worked the magic and, with that part of us that didn't really want to grow up; we believe that food somehow has the power to change our lives. That 'part' is just a subconscious program that can be disconnected or changed.

Love has the power to change our lives and that is what we really want when we crave food to heal negative emotions. But in the simple world of our childhood all we remember deep within our subconscious is that food=happiness. We forget the love it came with and just remember the feeling, and in just the same way that Pavlov's dogs salivated at the sound of the bell, even though there was no food, we expect that love will come with the food and so we just eat and eat and eat until we feel like bursting and then seem surprised that we feel sick instead of better, and so we eat some more because we know that trying harder is good. And we forget the power of simple distraction and the ease of a child's releasing of negative feelings, and just know that we'll feel better if we eat.

So what happens to us as adults, having learned, as children, that food is intimately connected with feeling better and being good?

If we have developed an unhealthy relationship with food, then whenever we are feeling a little down, a little fed-up, or maybe even just feeling a little restless – there is a strong temptation to head for the kitchen and find something to eat.

The something we find to eat is almost never an apple, a pear, a banana, a peach, a handful of grapes or dried fruit.

And the really interesting thing is that ten minutes after it's been eaten – the uncomfortable emotion is still there, only this time, as I mentioned earlier, it's tinged with guilt over having eaten, and guilt at having failed once more. So we spend the evening either battling the desire to eat more, or, desperately seeking love, we eat again... and again... and again...

Michael Hadfield

15. Love Is…

- Feeling alive.

- Feeling it matters that you exist.

- Feeling valued in your World.

- Being content with who you are.

- Recognising that you are worth the effort.

I need to be clear. When I use the word love I am not talking about intimacy or sex. I'm talking about feeling valued and important. I'm talking about knowing that someone cares that you exist. I'm talking about knowing that someone cares about how you feel. And I'm talking about feeling supported and encouraged, by those close to you, in your journey through life.

Oh I know that all sounds a bit like it's down to other people and, therefore, outside of your control, but the easier and more gentle you are with you; the more supporting and encouraging you are with you; the more you will find that others in your world begin to reflect this back to you. You have to make the first move. Then, as you love yourself more, not only will you lose weight because you've stopped hating your overweight body, but you will also find that life becomes easier and the World supports you more and more with your intentions, dreams and desires.

Michael Hadfield

16. Small Steps

So what steps do you need to take to change all this?

How do you start this process of taking back control of your life, and of your eating, in a way that is satisfying to you?

To begin with - whenever you have the desire to eat when it is not mealtime…

Make a note of what you are feeling on a scale.

$$0…1…2…3…4…5…6…7…8…9…10$$

0 is feeling good. 10 is feeling miserable.

Then eat whatever you want

10 minutes later check how you feel

Bloated…uncomfortable…not nice full…nice full…comfortable…nothing…empty

Train yourself into the new habit of noticing whatever feelings or emotions are present whenever you get the urge to eat – especially when you are planning to snack and going through that mental should I, shouldn't I, which we all know is going to end with you giving in to the urge, so why not save yourself the hassle and just eat.

Buy yourself a little notebook that's easy to keep to hand and just make a note of the date and time and the feeling or emotion. Imagine that scale from 0 to 10 where 0 is peaceful and happy and 10 is very distressed. Score the intensity of the feeling that's driving you to eat somewhere along that scale. Then go and eat, write down what you've eaten and ten minutes later score the feeling again. Also make a note of how comfortable your stomach feels. Score it bloated, uncomfortable, unpleasantly full, pleasantly full, comfortable, no sensations, empty.

If you find it easier, I've designed a diary sheet for this and you'll find a link where you can download it below.

www.HypnosisIsEasy.com/weight-loss-food-diary.htm

This food diary is just an information gathering exercise to begin the process of losing weight without dieting. This is not in any way designed to stop you enjoying your snacks. I encourage you to continue to enjoy your snacks – but only after completing your diary entry. If you allow me to help you and follow my guidance you may be surprised to find that your eating habits are changing comfortably and naturally and that your excess weight just starts to slip away.

17. Oh! yes… those Biscuits

In case you were still wondering about the relevance of that story about the biscuits – it contains a very important message that is a crucial part of the Diet-Free Weight Loss System.

But first I need to tell you about something else – something surprising that I remember reading about.

I came across it when I was exploring methods of using hypnosis to treat pain and physical diseases like cancer. I was following Google threads about pain research and came across an interesting piece about morphine use in hospitals. Morphine is never prescribed lightly, as it is an opium derivative and highly addictive.

Anyway some researchers decided to do a study on morphine use in hospitals.

What they found out was very surprising. It seems that a patient who is allowed to medicate herself with morphine (so she is totally in control of its administration) requires significantly less morphine to control her pain than a patient who is totally dependent on the doctor to decide amount and frequency. Isn't that fascinating? I found it interesting on two points. The first because it supported the idea I was exploring of pain being able to be influenced by thought, and the second was that knowing relief is available whenever you want it actually frees something up so that less pain is experienced.

And this really does relate to the biscuits.

When you have an unlimited supply and there are no restrictions on use, you not only use much less than when there is a limited supply and there are use restrictions, but you also need much less – the desire is reduced also.

It is the reduction of desire that is one of the keys. An easy way to reduce desire is to have no restrictions, no limits on what you can and can't have. You see part of our desire is because we've been taught that certain foods are special - maybe high-priced foods with exotic ingredients, foods for special occasions, or just *to make us feel better* when we are a little down.

Remove that and there is nothing left to drive the need to eat unnecessarily.

18. Obesity

"Many cultures throughout history have viewed obesity as the result of a character flaw. The *obesus* or fat character in Greek comedy was a glutton and figure of mockery. During Christian times food was viewed as a gateway to the sins of sloth and lust. In modern Western culture, excess weight is often regarded as unattractive, and obesity is commonly associated with various negative stereotypes. People of all ages can face social stigmatization, and may be targeted by bullies or shunned by their peers. Obesity is once again a reason for discrimination."

Wikipaedia

Obesity and Overweight are different. To find out which applies to you, you need to know your Body Mass Index (BMI). If you don't know your BMI there's a handy calculator on my web page at

www.HypnosisIsEasy.com/weight.htm

just type in your height and weight and it will tell you your BMI.

A BMI of between 25 and 30 is Overweight. A BMI of 30 or over is Obese.

For example: I'm just under 6ft and 172 lbs at the moment with a BMI of 24 which is ok. For someone 5' 9", 124 lbs is underweight, 125 - 168 lbs is ok, 169 - 202 lbs is

Overweight, and 203 lbs or over is Obese. Obesity brings with it many more health risks than just being overweight so if you fall into this category it might be an idea to think about making a decision to take action now. Action can be as simple as parking your car further away from where you want to go; spending an hour cooking something fresh rather than poking holes in some cellophane and sticking it in the microwave; walking for your paper rather than driving; putting half a spoon less sugar in your coffee; or leaving one tiny piece of something on your plate to be thrown away.

The action you take now doesn't need to be huge. It just needs to be a demonstration *to you* that you are willing to make changes, and small changes are so much easier to make than big changes. And so what if it takes you a year to lose 50lbs, your friend who loses 20 lbs in three weeks by starving herself will be doing the same thing again next year and finding it even harder, and again the year after that and finding it harder still. You won't. You won't because the actions you take are sustainable and lead to long-term permanent weight loss.

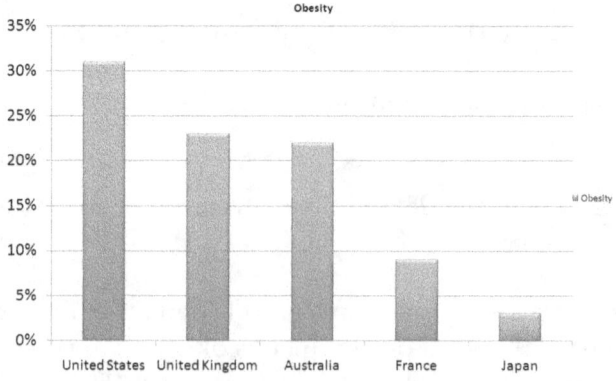

Obesity is a huge problem in the US and the UK. Here are a few facts & figures so you can see the size of it.

1971 – 2000 (US)

Obesity up from 14.5% - 30.9%

Energy (i.e. Calories) consumed 1971 – 2004 (US)

Women increased by 335 kCals/day

Men increased by 168 kCals/day

Most of this increase came from sweetened beverages and potato chips/crisps.

An amazing 25% of daily Calorie intake in young people today is from sweetened beverages, while childhood obesity rates are closely linked to TV watching. But that shouldn't really be any surprise. If you go out and run around and play you are bound to be fitter and slimmer than if you only exercise your thumb muscles playing video games.

Between 1977 and 1995 fast food sales tripled, but energy intake quadrupled.

Another significant factor is that obese people consistently under-report their food consumption compared to normalweights. This isn't about lying. People who are obese are just unaware of much of the food they consume. This is why that *Food Diary* is so important.

People who keep a food diary lose twice as much weight as those who don't.

But the good news is that since you aren't aware of much of the food you eat - you won't miss it.

Now it's time to have a look at the Big Lie you've been told and that has led you into the trap you find yourself where, no matter how hard you try, or how good you've been, you just end up - sooner or later - heavier than you were before.

19. The Big Lie

This is the Science bit (like they do in the hair adverts) it's important and it won't last long so stay with me.

The first source to which the body turns for energy is something called glycogen. Glycogen is a complex carbohydrate that is stored in the body. 65% of it is stored in skeletal muscles; the rest is in the liver. So when the body is short of calories (which is a circumstance that diets are designed to create) it gets the missing calories from muscle tissue and the liver.

When glycogen is nearly depleted, then, and only then, does the body turn to metabolise fat stores in fatty tissue. At this point you've lost a great deal of muscle and probably shrunk your liver.

Because muscle is very much denser than fat you clearly lose weight, but body shape doesn't change quickly because there is not much loss of volume. And let's face it, changing body shape is the reason most of us diet. If we all weighed 300lbs but looked fantastic no one would bother trying to lose weight.

So remember…

Dieting burns muscle not fat.

Michael Hadfield

20. Tried and Failed?

Research clearly shows that...

Diets don't work better the more you do them.

There is no significant difference between diets.

Dieting can seriously damage your health.

Most of the people who come to me for help with controlling their weight have tried diets – and failed. Sometimes they've tried diets on several occasions and still failed. Many of them have been members of WeightWatchers or Slimming World and still they end up in my consulting room wanting to lose weight.

Now it's not that these activities don't help you lose weight. They do. If you cut down your food intake sufficiently anyone can lose weight.

Don't eat – you lose weight. No question about that.

What you find though is that reaching the target weight is a real struggle, and also unsustainable. I once saw a picture of one of the weight clubs Slimmer of the Year taken ten years ago looking gorgeous and a current photo of her heavier than she ever has been in her life. It's just that the weight clubs don't advertise that.

The problem is not that you can't lose weight with these methods – you can. The problem is that you cannot keep it off. I need to make it clear that I am not knocking these methods. A very good friend of mine was very successful at running several Slimming World Groups and I know how hard she worked and how much she was driven by wanting to make a positive difference in people's lives. I also know many of the people who attended her groups and they had nothing but praise for her. The events were fun and laughter filled.

But I also know that these people could not keep the weight off. They could follow the guidelines and enjoy their Syns for only so long before giving in to what they considered 'normal' eating.

Then spring would turn up again (like it does every year), or a wedding, or other predictable social event and so they would return to the fold, and the public weighing, and get back on the treadmill for a while. It's a great social event. It helps with weight loss short-term. And if that's what you want then I highly recommend it. It just won't solve your weight problem permanently.

If short-term fast weight loss is what you want then what I am offering isn't for you. If you want to put an end to all this dieting nonsense and lose weight in a way that is sustainable then stay with me.

21. This is What I am Offering You

What I'm describing here is a healthy relationship with food, sustainable weight loss, and an easy way to lose weight without food restrictions.

What I'm also giving you is the opportunity to make a choice to lose weight, keep it off, and change your relationship with food so that your excess weight will gently disappear (giving your skin more time to adapt to the changes). Diets only deal with food at the Calorie, or Carbohydrate, or Sugar, or Fat, level. All they do is get you thinking about what you eat and your whole life starts to revolve around food – and not in a good way – simply because what you used to eat is largely off-limits.

Sustainable change is built slowly and steadily from small changes.

Diets require large changes in eating patterns and habits.

But the kicker is this. Diets do nothing about your relationship with food. Diets do nothing about your beliefs about food. Diets do nothing about your subconscious needs and desires. They just leave you with a battle.

A battle you can't win.

With Diet-free Weight Loss you can eat what you want when you want and still lose weight.

Michael Hadfield

22. Metabolism Myth Buster

Metabolism is another one of those words that gets bandied about a lot in weight loss circles. I've discovered that there's a whole lot of hokey about metabolism in connection with losing weight and dieting.

Here's the Truth.

Eating less *slows* metabolism. Because of the food shortage your body thinks famine so it *makes fat*. Metabolism slows, because a slower metabolic rate burns less fuel so the fuel you've got lasts longer - this is an essential survival mechanism for when food is scarce. Then when normal eating resumes your slowed metabolism means more food turned to fat rather than burned.

Metabolism is your body's engine. It burns fuel – but it has an intelligent accelerator. When the tank is constantly running near empty, and filling stations seem few and far between, it runs slower and if you do that to it often enough, it learns, and ends up running permanently in conservation mode - making it ever harder to shift those excess pounds.

Michael Hadfield

23. Moody Blues

Mood states are, I believe, of much greater significance than Calorie intake when it comes to losing weight.

So consider...

Weight is an emotional problem.

Diet results in social isolation.

Social isolation = low mood.

Low mood = comfort eating.

Mood is a much bigger factor than food. In other words it's not so much the calories you eat as the reason you eat them.

If your friends are largely overweight then success at losing weight will produce social pressure to 'give in' and 'have a little bit of this, a little bit won't do you any harm' from those who are not able to control their eating - just do them a favour and pass on this book. If nothing else it will stop their sabotage attempts.

At the subconscious level self-sabotage results from the feeling that you will no longer be part of the fat club and end up without friends. This is also a problem with social weight loss groups like Weight Watchers, Jenny Craig, and Slimming World. Reaching your target weight means you are out of the club, you lose friends and social activity – powerful subconscious reasons to keep on sabotaging your attempts to lose weight.

The trick is to find other solutions to low mood states – solutions that help you to feel much better than the food does. You don't need to comfort eat when you have available other simple and easy strategies to increase your comfort. If you decide to buy my set of CDs to help support you in your weight loss program then I also include with them ideas and strategies you can use to improve your mood.

No one else gets to live *your* life. Your life is for you to make of it what you will. So make it the best life you know how to, and if others don't like that then it's just tough. As long as you allow yourself to be influenced and manipulated by others - they are the ones living your life, not you. So choose to be slimmer, and choose to make your own choices.

24. Waste or Waist

You know what the one thing that all weight loss clients have in common when they first come to see me? Not one of them can throw food away. Even if they feel full half way through a big meal they will plough on until the plate is cleaned. Then they'll find room for dessert.

If you do nothing else but overcome this challenge you will start to lose weight immediately.

When I think back to my last junior school (I went to four different junior schools), when I was about 9, I have a vivid memory of a child sitting opposite me being chided by the dinner lady for not clearing their plate. They were told in no uncertain terms that there would be no dessert for them, unless they cleaned their plate. Starving children in Africa were mentioned and they were supposed to be grateful for what they received. The meals were pretty much overcooked slop, delivered in a van from somewhere, because the school had no cooking facilities of its own, just a kitchen to serve meals and wash dishes. I felt that it was most unfair to be 'made' to eat something that you didn't like.

I was lucky, my Mum was a good cook, so I never had a problem eating everything at home, and it was such a pleasant change from school food. The thought of 'wasting' any of it never entered my head. But I was aware of this culture that said that wasting food was a bad thing to do and Mum would often tell us stories of how fortunate we were because during the War (WWII) all luxury foods and a lot of staples were rationed and even something as straightforward as having as much butter as I wanted would be impossible when you were only allowed 2oz of the stuff a week.

So, as I was growing up, I was growing up alongside a whole generation whose parents had suffered serious food hardship. For them waste was a legitimate crime because they recognized the absolute luxury of having plenty to eat. Like all good parents, they wanted to ensure that their children would never go hungry in the way they had been.

Then around 1964 one of my teachers got us involved in collecting money for famine relief and the TV news was full of horrific pictures of swollen bellied malnourished children. These things make a powerful impact on young minds. This is especially true when parents then use these horrific images to lovingly 'blackmail' us into eating everything up 'because there are starving children in Africa who would be glad of that'. What sensitive child would want anyone to starve because she hadn't cleaned her plate?

Then, of course, we all grew up, programmed with these ideas about it being a terrible sin to waste food, and proceeded to program our own children with the same ideas, though I seem to remember insisting on cleaning plates largely because it was the healthy stuff that was being wasted. I modified the exhortation to eat up and simply pointed out that if they couldn't finish it 'they must be full' and so 'you won't want any dessert'. I just didn't want them living on sugars and fats, but it makes no difference what the rationale is, *encouraging* children to *eat up* does them no favours.

If cleaning your plate is heavily programmed into you, here's what you do.

Recognise now that it is just a program that is running within you and making choices for you that are not your choices. They are someone else's choices. When we attempt to 'defy' one of these subconscious programs we get an emotional reaction - in this case very likely a feeling of guilt, but whatever it is, we feel uncomfortable. The only way, in the past, we knew how to get rid of this emotional discomfort was to do what it was telling us to do.

I'm going to let you into a little secret. An uncomfortable feeling is just that - a feeling. It doesn't mean you are bad. It doesn't mean you are doing anything wrong. It just means there's an old program running. You can safely ignore the discomfort. Just allow it be there. In fact you could even welcome it and invite it to do its worst. If you are courageous enough to do that you'll find that the feeling very rapidly dissipates and is replaced by warm feelings of accomplishment and success.

Next time you have a meal leave one pea, one chip, one small piece of anything on the plate. When you scrape it into the bin, feel good about those calories that are not now settling down as fat cells somewhere in your body. Then, next time you sit down to enjoy a meal remember that the wasted pea caused no terrible catastrophe. Nobody starved who wasn't already starving. No ill befell you. In fact you can allow yourself to feel really pleased because that was probably the single most-difficult step you have to take on this journey towards a slimmer, fitter, healthier you. But leave two peas, two chips, one bit each of two different things next time.

Repeat this for several days, each time wasting a little bit more of something that is of no consequence. Once you realize you can get away with wasting a little food you are ready for the next step.

While you are eating be mindful of how full/hungry you feel. Notice how the hunger dissipates almost as soon as you start your meal. Then a little bit later the full sensations start to make their presence felt. As soon as you feel comfortably full STOP EATING and throw the rest in the bin - no matter how much is left on your plate.

Comfortably full is when you have no discomfort moving around and you feel satisfied (though satisfaction is also affected by the quality of the food you eat - sugar & fat can fill you without any sense of satisfaction so they leave you wanting more even if you are bloated.

As soon as you start to feel that full feeling, STOP EATING take a moment and then look at what's left on your plate. This 'moment' is really important because it disconnects you from the plate of food and allows you to see it for what it is. Notice how the liquids congeal as they cool, the mess you've made moving stuff around on the plate, and ask yourself - if I was presented with this, just the way it is right now, would I want to eat it or would I be repulsed? See it as if it's someone else's leftovers.

Then just do whatever you want to do. But know that if you continue to eat, every mouthful will feel a little more difficult to swallow because you know the truth now and the truth, as they say, is trying to set you free and allow you to be that slimmer person that you wish to be.

It's okay to stop eating when your body sends you its full message.

As you continue to practice this you will discover that you have been putting far too much food on your plate, so you will start serving yourself smaller portions. Buy yourself a slightly smaller plate, that way your eyes will be telling the remnants of that old program that you are still eating loads of food.

If you follow none of my advice, apart from wasting food, you will lose weight. Learn how to do this and you will be free to make your own choices and you will find that other healthy changes to your eating patterns just happen naturally and spontaneously.

Michael Hadfield

25. You Won't Miss This

I've told you that diets don't work. I've told you to waste food. I've told you that you can eat what you want and still lose weight. But we both know that there's something else has to happen too. There is one other place where we can make small changes and produce big results.

In the chapter on Obesity I mentioned food diaries and how people who are obese are not aware of much of what they eat. This isn't just true of people who are obese. It's true of anyone who has an unhealthy relationship with food. I've also mentioned subconscious, or hidden, programs that control eating patterns. I'd like to look at another aspect of subconscious programs.

But first I need to digress a little.

If you drive, you'll remember the very first time you sat behind the steering wheel and had to take the car out on the road with other cars. Do you remember how impossible it all seemed? All the things you had to do at the same time - watch behind, watch in front, all the controls and the pedals, watch the traffic signals, watch other motorists and do all that without hitting anything and still steer in a straight line? Now, do you give any of that a thought? In fact you probably give it so little thought that on occasion you've found yourself somewhere you didn't intend to be because you were daydreaming and the 'driving program' in you just took you where you normally go.

That ability to drive without apparently giving the task of driving any attention is because the driving program has it all on automatic so you only need to pay attention when a problem crops up that the driving program doesn't have a subroutine to handle.

Eating is like that. It's so automatic that we pay little attention to it. When we are hungry we pay attention to food and we savour the first few mouthfuls, but after that we barely notice what we are chewing and swallowing. When we eat habitually during TV breaks, or coffee breaks, the food itself is rarely noticed because the eating itself is just *something to do*.

So consider that if you are eating with just a barely peripheral awareness of the food, you'd hardly notice if you weren't doing it, but were engaged in some other activity instead.

This unnoticed food is where you can lose a lot of calories from your daily diet without any suffering or sense of deprivation. This is where your biggest change can take place while still leaving you to eat what you want when you want. Make a commitment to yourself to eat consciously and enjoy everything you eat. Eat slowly, and if you can wean yourself off reading or watching TV while you eat so much the better. Concentrate on all the flavours, and textures - the whole experience of eating. Eat slowly and enjoy rather than be planning the next forkful to shovel into your mouth.

When you eat this way you will very quickly realize that most of your pleasure comes from the first few mouthfuls and it dissipates after that. Learn to notice the point at which the pleasure has gone and you have shifted into your habitual programmed eating 'just because it's there'. This is the point at which to stop eating. Nothing is lost at this point. You've had all the pleasure. You've had the satisfaction. Further eating is pointless.

The beauty of eating like this is not only that you lose weight, but also that, just because you feel full and stop eating or stop eating because the pleasure has gone, you can eat again any time the hunger returns and the pleasure is once more available to experience. I frequently eat dessert now anything from two to four hours after the main meal. After the main meal I'm satisfied. But I really enjoy dessert so I wait and if I feel hungry again later in the evening I have some, and if I don't I don't. I haven't made up a rule saying I shouldn't eat dessert because it's all sugar and flour and fat and I want to lose weight. I've made up a rule saying I'll have it when I know I'm going to enjoy it, and I won't have it when I'm already full. This attitude towards food is incredibly freeing because it creates none of the resistance that diets create so there is nothing to kick up against and food rapidly becomes a non-issue.

I used to love chocolate. Now I find milk chocolate so sickly sweet that I can't stand it in my mouth and I only eat plain chocolate. When I have a bar of plain chocolate I'll eat one or two squares because after that there is no pleasure so eating more would be pointless. I can have a bar in the fridge now for several weeks at a time, eating only one or two squares when I feel in the mood. This happened quite naturally and effortlessly as I followed my own rules.

There is just one more thing I want to touch on before I start to wrap things up.

This is something I've called Healthy Hunger.

I've come across quite a few people who seem to be afraid of being hungry. Have you ever heard anyone say something like 'I'll eat now in case I don't get a chance later'? People avoid that hungry feeling. They've come to believe that somehow they should never feel like that. Mind you, they choose to smother lots of other emotions with food, so it might just be a question of somehow having learned that they don't like to feel and would rather live as some sort of emotionless zombie.

It's no way to live. Feelings (good and bad) are a part of being human and let us know we're alive. Hunger is just one of them. Hunger is nature's way of saying 'time to go and kill something for dinner'. So you pick up your spears and arrows, get together with your mates and head off to return many hours later with a wonderful appetite (Healthy Hunger) only to then have to wait while dinner is gutted, skinned, and roasted. Or if you're on the gathering side, rather than the hunting side of things, then hunger is go and find some berries and roots and fruits. Again this takes several hours, and again requires lengthy preparation of the food. If we didn't have that hunger feeling we'd just laze around all day in our hammocks in the jungle. It's what gets us moving and gives us the exercise we need to stay healthy.

Now consider modern Western life.

Slightest twinge of hunger, or even the thought that if I don't do something I'll get hungry and I'd better make sure that doesn't happen. So, quick trip to the kitchen (or at the very worst supermarket), then open packet, and pop complete meal into oven or microwave. Reducing this to its most ridiculous it's a case of boil kettle and pour hot water onto dehydrated pasta, wait a couple of minutes and then mix in chemical flavour (because it doesn't have any) and enjoy crunchy peas with powdery middles. Bodies were designed to eat several hours after the hunger feeling started, but we've got that down to about 30 minutes, or less. Or in the case of snacks rather than meals the food is in the mouth almost before we've even thought about what to eat.

I like feeling that feeling of healthy hunger. It tells me I'm going to enjoy the food so much more than when I eat without feeling that feeling. In fact writing all this has got that feeling going in me right now and it's going to be several hours before I eat and I'm going to cook something that takes 90 minutes in the oven and half an hour of preparation and it's going to be delicious because I'm going to be feeling ready for it by the time I eat later on.

Learn to cultivate that feeling of Healthy Hunger and enjoy it.

Michael Hadfield

26. Getting Started

I've given you all this information on how to lose weight easily and free yourself from diets forever so that you understand the ways in which you have been manipulated into following someone else's agenda. I've also given you lots of suggestions as to how you can go about putting all of this into practice in your life. But as a therapist I discovered that knowing why something is the way it is, and knowing what steps to take, doesn't do a single thing to change it, but that knowledge does act as a lubricant making the subsequent change process so much easier - when you decide to take action.

So now it's up to you. Make a choice, right now, to be slimmer and to develop a healthy, sustainable relationship with food.

So to summarise, here's the 10 steps you have to take to start losing those excess pounds.

1. Let yourself off the hook for being overweight. You are the way you are. The past is gone and there isn't a single thing you can do to change anything that's already happened - no matter how much you want to. What you can do is make a decision, right this instant, that you are going to become whatever weight or size you've decided, and that this is your first step in learning how to be in control and have the same sort of relationship with food that slimmer people have.

2. Weigh yourself and write down your weight and your BMI (using the calculator). This is just so you can be pleased with your progress and make a commitment to yourself that you will never again be that heavy. Then weigh yourself just once a week if you feel this will motivate you and keep you on track. If ups and downs in your weight will demoralise you then don't do this, but make sure you do all the other stuff. It will take longer to notice your clothes becoming looser so just make the changes, enjoy your food and expect results.

3. Start a food diary and keep track of what you are eating.

4. Throw food away.

5. Eat only when you feel hungry and even then not immediately.

6. Stop eating when the pleasure has gone or you notice you are starting to feel full.

7. If you want to eat, then eat, but stop when you've had enough - even if you find you've had enough after just one mouthful. Frequently the desire is completely satisfied with just one taste. Anyway most of the desire comes from knowing you shouldn't and wanting to kick against this.

8. Keep your weight loss intentions to yourself. This makes it much more difficult for others to sabotage your efforts and you won't feel any pressure to supply progress reports. You'll find that this makes it much easier to lose weight slowly, gently and permanently. If

others notice a change in your eating habits all you have to do is say I'm not feeling hungry right now, or I'm feeling really full, in order to escape any pressure to eat more than you have decided to.

9. Make sure you eat breakfast - even if it's only a little bit. From evening meal to lunchtime is effectively a 'food is in short supply' message. If you eat breakfast you are less likely to snack and will be hungry again by lunchtime. Coffee and donuts is not what I've got in mind though.

10. You must exercise. Now, before you switch off, I'm not saying you must go to the gym. I'm not saying you've got to drive yourself round the bend with boredom by pounding a treadmill for an hour a day. For exercise to be effective you must enjoy it. If you don't enjoy it you will eventually find excuses to stop doing it. The excuses will get more frequent, the weight loss will slow, you'll think it's all a waste of time again and give up. Fit muscle burns calories even while it is resting. I usually manage to walk between 2 and 3 miles a day on at least 5 days of the week. Even on those occasions when I don't really want to I always feel so much better when I get back. And now that I've been doing that for so long that it's become a habit I find that I get the uncomfortable feelings when I'm prevented from going out. So it's good to develop beneficial habits. If you aren't a fan of exercise think in terms of walking, cycling, swimming, dancing, or a beginner's exercise class to get you started and see how it goes. Try it a few times, if you don't like it try something else. I even use exercise DVDs in the winter when the weather makes it more difficult to

get outside. Doing a little you enjoy is better than doing a lot that you hate.

Now you know how you've been misled. You can see how diets are a waste of time and how it is so much better for your physical and mental health to take a longer-term approach. There are huge benefits to simply maintaining a healthy weight. So make the healthy choice, rather than mistreating your body by over-eating and then dieting all your muscle away in a desperate attempt to return to a body shape that pleases you.

So here's what you need to do now…

27. What Next?

I hope you've enjoyed this book and found it valuable. I really hope that it's given you some insight into why you have always failed to lose weight permanently and some really helpful tips, like the food diary.

But there's more to losing weight than knowing why it's difficult. Knowing why it's difficult, and knowing the traps that others have led you into, is just the beginning of your journey towards a slimmer healthier more attractive body.

Now it's time to take action.

Have another look at that 10-step action list in the previous chapter. If you want to take it really easy and literally step-by-step then start now with step 1 (that's easy and is really just a thought experiment). Tomorrow look at step 2 and so on. But make sure you look at that list every day just to remind yourself what needs to be done.

But I can do a lot more for you.

The information that I've given you in this book is sufficient for you to make all the changes that you need to make. But I know that some people read self-help books, think 'hey! that was great' and immediately start looking for the next book.

Losing weight is something you have to engage with. Reading the right book can be incredibly helpful but you need to take action. Now I know that the action bit is the most difficult and if you are someone who likes things to be just as easy as they can be then I can help you with that too.

I've mentioned earlier in this book that I'm a therapist who helps people with weight loss and other psychological and health problems. I mostly use hypnosis to help people make those changes. You remember I talked about those subconscious programs that cause you to eat without awareness, or carry on eating when you are full? Well hypnosis is the quickest, easiest way I know to change those subconscious programs so they do something more useful than screwing your life up. That's not to say you can't change them yourself - you can, it just takes longer, and unfortunately we live in a society where people want quick results - which is one of the reasons why this weight loss process will not be popular with a lot of people because it doesn't promise instant results.

What you get instead is lasting results.

So what I've done for you, just to make this whole process of changing your eating patterns, and forming a healthy relationship with food, easier, is to create a set of 3 CDs to support you in this process. But I don't want to get into a sales pitch. I just want to make sure you know that they are available if you need them. If you want to make this process of losing weight as easy and effortless as possible then visit

www.HypnosisIsEasy.com/how-to-lose-weight-easily-cds.htm

and make your purchase. There are more details about the CDs and how they will help you to lose weight on the above web page.

Here's what one of my customers has to say about my CD-based weight loss program.

"It's really really good!!! And I'm 13lbs down!!!! I really do think it's brilliant!!! I just thought you should know that I appreciate it and use it. I'd go as far as saying anyone that is struggling to shift weight!! Try it!!! It's the best.... And trust me I've tried a few!!!!"

Janet Whitfield

Michael Hadfield

Appendix

Personality Profile?

As a therapist I get to notice patterns that occur in people who come to me for help with similar problems. These are either behavioural patterns or beliefs about how their world works. I usually find that making small changes to behaviours or beliefs frequently produces results that are completely out of proportion to the size of the change.

Here are some of the patterns that I've noticed seem to be associated with weight problems. It's a big list but have a read through it and see just how much of it matches with you.

- They are overweight. Anything from 20lbs to 100lbs, though most want to lose around 30lbs to 40lbs.

- They generally don't like their job, or they like their job but the boss, or one or two colleagues, create a stressful environment.

- They generally spend most evenings watching TV.

- Exercise is something they are planning on doing.

- They don't throw food away – however much is on the plate gets eaten.

- Several attempts at dieting.

- They snack on chocolate, crisps (potato chips), biscuits (cookies), cake, and bread – with other stuff added to the bread.

- They believe they have no will power.

- They eat regardless of whether or not they are hungry.

- Low mood state (I include boredom here) triggers eating more often than not.

- Commercial breaks generally control when and what to eat (chair-kitchen-get food-chair) has to be complete before the program restarts.

- About 1 in 3 have been to Slimming World or Weight Watchers.

- Many see themselves as failures.

- They feel out of control.

- Many appear unfulfilled in life.

- Some have emotional issues around food from childhood.

- Some have other emotional issues around childhood.

- About half of them are in unsatisfactory relationships.

- They generally don't want a quick fix, they want sustainable weight loss – even if it takes a while.

- They want something that works.

- For all of them I am a last resort.

Michael Hadfield

Connect with me online:

You can find out a little bit more about me, Michael Hadfield, here:

www.HypnosisIsEasy.com/bio.htm

Website: **www.HypnosisIsEasy.com**

Twitter: @m_hadfield

Facebook: Hypnosis is Easy

My blog: **http://HypnosisIsEasy.com/wordpress/**

Or if you prefer you can find all the links mentioned in this book here:

www.HypnosisIsEasy.com/howto

If you enjoyed this book and found my information helpful to you then please be sure to let me know by leaving a comment on the above web page. If you have any weight loss issues that you'd like me to address, then again please leave me a comment on the above web page. Your feedback is important to me and will help to guide me with future projects.

####

www.ingramcontent.com/pod-product-compliance
Lightning Source LLC
Chambersburg PA
CBHW071325310526
45789CB00016B/920